MW00939797

Ayurveda

Ayurvedic Essential Oils & Aromatherapy for Amazing Relaxation, Beautiful Skin and Tremendous Healing

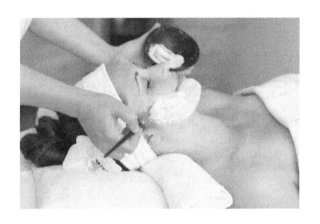

By James Adler and Elena Garcia

Copyright James Adler and Elena Garcia©

2014, 2016

All rights reserved. No part of this publication may be reproduced, stored in a retrieval system, or transmitted, in any form or by any means, electronic, mechanical, photocopying, recording or otherwise, without the prior written permission of the author and the publishers.

The scanning, uploading, and distribution of this book via the Internet or via any other means without the permission of the author is illegal and punishable by law. Please purchase only authorized electronic editions, and do not participate in or encourage electronic piracy of copyrighted materials.

Disclaimer:

A physician has not written the information in this book. Although Ayurvedic therapies are generally safe to use, if you suffer from any serious medical condition, are pregnant, or on medication you should consult your doctor (preferably a doctor who specializes in oriental medicine) first to see if you can apply it. It is also advisable that you visit a qualified Ayurvedic Doctor so that you can obtain a highly personalized treatment for your case, especially if you want to make Ayurveda a part of your lifestyle. This book is for informational and educational purposes only.

All information in this book has been carefully researched and checked for factual accuracy. However, the author and publishers make no warranty, expressed or implied, that the information contained herein is appropriate for every individual, situation or purpose, and assume no responsibility for errors or omission. The reader assumes the risk and full responsibility for all actions, and the author will not be held liable for any loss or damage, whether consequential, incidental, and special or otherwise that may result from the information presented in this publication.

If you are pregnant or have any serious health condition, do not use any aromatherapy treatments described in this book without consulting with your physician and aromatherapy practitioner first.

"Self massage with aromatherapy ignites your internal pharmacy, and stimulates all the systems of your body"
Deepak Chopra

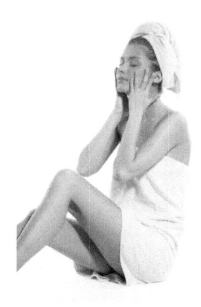

TABLE OF CONTENTS:

Free Complimentary PDF eBook
from Elena & James

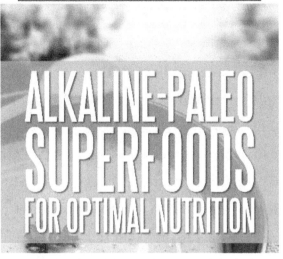

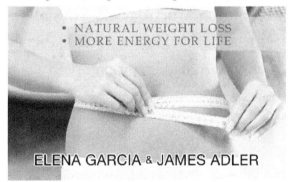

Download link:

www.bitly.com/alkapaleofree

Introduction to Aromatherapy and the Ayurvedic Lifestyle

Thanks for purchasing our book. We are Elena and James, a married couple interested in holistic health and oriental therapies. A few years ago we decided to immerse ourselves in the amazing world of Ayurveda (the traditional natural medicine that originated in India about 5000 years ago). We first went on a month long vacation to India and traveled the country. We got really interested in the food, the culture, and their methods of healing. James had done his basic introductory training in Ayurveda before (he is a health coach and a life coach), but for me, Elena, it was like a new discovery. We like our Western aromatherapy, but Ayurveda makes it much more holistic.

We have decided to put this booklet together to share our passion for Ayurvedic Wellness with you and to show how easy it is to incorporate some highly therapeutic healing rituals into your everyday life. We especially recommend this book for beginners in both aromatherapy and Ayurveda, but we also hope that if you are not new to those topics, you will also find some new tips, motivation and inspiration.

We stand by the belief that one thing is to know and another is to apply. This is the mistake that we have both done, for example, we knew so many great wellness tips from Ayurveda but we did not take any action to commit ourselves to it. Hence, sometimes the excess of knowledge does not equal to putting theory into practice. This is why we would like to encourage you to use this book to actually do your own Ayurvedic healing spa, meditate, relax and heal yourself and those around you on a regular basis.

Finally, we would like to add that we are not Ayurvedic doctors or gurus. We are here to spread the word of Ayurveda in a practical way. We believe that life is all about learning. Actually, the more we learn, the less we think we know! We are students of Ayurveda and will always be. This is a never ending story.

One of our Ayurveda teachers from Kerala used to say, "All those Westerners come here to learn some practical Ayurvedic solutions. They want to learn more about their own bodies and minds. They also want to know how to undo the damage that very often they have done to themselves by their fast-paced Western lifestyle. They tell me that I know a lot. To be honest,

I always tell them that I know very little. I am still learning from my master and I always tell him that he does know a lot. He, in turn replies that he does not know that much and it's his master who knows a lot and he looks up to...and so on and so forth..."

We hope that you understand what we mean by the learning process. This is what Ayurveda is all about; it is the science of life, getting to know yourself and even those around you. There are also emotions involved as well as your mental attitude; it's not only about the physical health. It's all interconnected.

As you probably already know, or heard, *Ayurveda* is essentially an ancient system of Hindu traditional medicine native to India. It originated as an extension of the *Rigveda*, contrary to some beliefs where it is seen as a part of *Atharva-Veda*. *Charaksamhita* and *Susrutha Samhita* are the oldest and foundational Ayurvedic texts.

Ayurveda approaches the enumeration of our body in 5 typical elements, also known as the P*anchabhuta*. These 5 elements are:

- Fire (Agni)
- Air (Vayu)
- Water (Jal)
- Ether (Akasha)
- Earth (Prithvi)

Ayurveda also has 7 classic tissues, also known as D*hatu*, which are:

- Plasma or *rasa,*
- Blood or *rakta,*
- Muscles or *masa,*
- Fat or *meda*, bone or *asthi,*
- Semen or shukra and
- Marrow or majja

This system of medicine follows the principle of maintaining a balance in the three humors, or doshas, as they are called.

This balance means a state of health, in contrast to imbalance, which is suggestive of a disease or a disorder. Notice that our modern, Western medicine does not include this concept, as it assumes that you are perfectly healthy if there are not any symptoms visible and that you are ill when the diseases manifests itself. Then, of course, our Western doctors prescribe something that is supposed to kill the symptoms, but very often causes havoc and imbalances to the rest of the organs.

The oriental medicine is more about being persistent in observing one's body and making it one's goals to take good care of oneself. Ayurveda works with plenty of natural therapies ranging from balanced nutrition and herbs to aromatherapy and massage. There is also yoga and meditation.

Each natural therapy can be adopted in a different way according to your dosha type.

Let's have a look at Ayurvedic Doshas, this step of getting to know ayurveda is like getting to know yourself, your body, mind and emotions. This is a process where you just have to ask yourself dozens of questions, and you should also pay attention and observe your own body, something that we oftentimes neglect (Western standards of life are so awful!).

Various imbalances can arise out of lack or excess of either of the following humors or *Doshas*:

- **Vata-** This belongs to the idea of the 'impulse principle' or the nervous system.

- **Pitta-** This belongs to the transforming principle and primarily works according to the secretion of the bilious humor, which is crucial in direct digestion and metabolism. This humor essentially deals with the digestive system of the human body.

- **Kapha-** This is the body fluid principle which deals with mucous and its function in lubrication and nourishment.

Doshas are not like a visible concept that can be touched and easily categorized. We all consist of them, and one of them is our prevalent dosha. We are born with some kinds of predisposition, for example James is vata/pitta type and Elena is kapha type. In order to achieve balance, and therefore the ultimate wellness, one should know their prevalent dosha and learn how to use ayurvedic natural therapies and tailor them to their own needs. If you are a beginner, we know that it all may sound really complicated, but as they say: "different strokes for different folks" Makes total sense, right?

So, let's dive into the doshas, it's fun as you can try to figure out which one would be your prevalent dosha. Of course, to be 100% sure, you would need to book an appointment with an Ayurvedic doctor or practitioner so that they can diagnose you after asking you dozens of questions and doing some tests (again, it's fun, we really encourage you to play the doshas game!).

Vata- Vata people are thin, very often tall as well, and energetic. They have creative minds that ponder easily and they love new experiences like travelling and meeting new people. They are always on the go and doing something but they may also experience a sudden drop of energy. They oftentimes have cold feet and hands.

When unbalanced, they may experience constipation, headache, anxiety and insomnia. They don't benefit from irregular lifestyle patterns and they need to stick to their healthy routine like balanced meals, regular work shifts and sleep patterns. Vatas can get angry very easily. But they also know how to forgive and don't hold a grudge.

On the physical level, vata people normally have dry skin and dry, fragile hair.

Once the vata dosha is out of balance, the following conditions may manifest: lack of appetite, arthritis, weakness, and digestive problems.

Pitta- Pitta people are excellent leaders, they love being in charge. They are also very intellectual and are excellent decision makers (Vatas, on the other hand, are really creative but very often in two minds when it comes to making a decision).

Pittas can be short-tempered and always have to be right. They have strong digestion and so very often they think they can neglect their nutrition and eat whatever they want.

They are great speakers and know how to express themselves, they can often be too direct and so offend some people.

On the physical level, pitta people are usually of medium size /weight. They very often have ginger or red hair and fair complexion. They may be also prone to balding.

Unlike vatas, they always have warm hands and feet, this is why it is recommended they use cooling oils for self-massage.

Kapha- Kapha people have big bones and strong body. They have an excellent stamina but are characterized by such features as being slow, solid, steady and soft. They tend to be really calm and organized as well as supportive and helpful for other people. They like leading a peaceful and organized lifestyle and are not fond of changes, in fact it's hard for them to end a relationship or quit a job.

They also have tendency to accumulate old things at home (they love staying at home!) and are also prone to excess weight, water retention, depression, and very often stubbornness. They find it very difficult to take action so as to embark on something new.

They love to sleep excessively and to take naps.

An increase or decrease in any of these doshas shall lead to an imbalance. This imbalance is rectified by finding a *srota,* or the source of this alteration. This alteration is explained by Ayurveda as the lack of healthy channels for the smooth functioning of these humors. Aromatherapy massage oils, or *Swedana* (steam therapy) are just an examples of natural ayurvedic therapies used to bring balance.

Buddhism and Hinduism play a major role and have a major influence on the central principles of Ayurveda. An emphasis is given to balance whereas suppression of urges is unhealthy and can lead to sickness.

Here is a really funny example: when you suppress a sneeze, it can lead to shoulder pain. However, it also advocates that certain urges should be maintained in a reasonable manner, like moderate intake of food, adequate sleep and sexual intercourse.

Excess can be harmful, and so can be the lack of something. Westerners, when stressed out or confused, very often resort to alcohol, drugs and sex, but usually end up more stressed out and missing the balance. Ayurveda can help you learn more about you and prescribe a myriad of natural therapies that will make up the lack of certain dosha, but at the same time will reduce the possible excess of another dosha.

Practices derived from *Ayurveda* are a part of the Complementary and Alternative Medicine (CAM). This form of medicine is either complementary or alternative since it delineates itself from the conventional, scientific form of medicine. Along with Ayurveda, *Siddha* medicine and traditional Chinese medicine also form a part of Complementary and Alternative Medicine.

Aromatherapy, as a holistic therapy, takes into account the physical and the mental well being, along with lifestyle and eating habits. Coined by Frenchman Gaffoseer in 1936, this practice uses essential oils extracted from plants for the healing and therapeutic purposes. Aromatherapy may be considered a relatively new therapy in our Western culture, perhaps even a little bit over-hyped these days, but it has been used for ages and it forms an integral part of Ayurveda

This treatment involves addressing the imbalance in a patient, especially with respect to cognitive function, mood or mental health. This form of treatment is found to be useful in the treatment of various common complaints related to the respiratory system, the lymphatic system, circulation, skin, hair, and the nervous system.

In fact, aromatherapy has the capacity to slow down the sympathetic system, which is the system responsible for the fight or flight reaction and, at the same time, it stimulates the parasympathetic system, which is the one responsible for pleasant feelings and emotions. Hence, aromatherapy can have almost an immediate positive effect on your general well being.

According to Dr. Light Miller, of Ayurveda and Aromatherapy fame, a disease has 6 stages, which are defined as:
a) Accumulation
b) Aggravation
c) Dissemination
d) Relocation
e) Manifestation
f) Disruption

She asserts that imbalance can occur at the Accumulation stage due to improper lifestyle and eating habits. This is in contrast to the western idea of medicine, where the imbalance is acknowledged at the Manifestation stage.

Aromatherapy Massage

This branch of Aromatherapy is known as **Abhangaya,** which is a daily massage routine; it has also been practiced by Indian women for their infants for many years.

In India, new born babies are massaged with oils until the age of three, as it enhances circulation of blood, mobility of joints and builds their immune system. This has often been seen as a practice of the social rural culture.

I am sure you have heard of Indian head massage. If you ever go to India, make sure you treat yourself to it on a daily basis and experience how good it feels. So much better and real energy stimulating than our Western cup of coffee!

Of course, you don't have to go to India to try Indian head Massage; there are plenty of highly qualified practitioners in the Western countries, and thanks to this book, you will learn enough about Ayurvedic Aromatherapy to perform one at home whenever you need it!

The most famous Indian Head Massage guru is Narenda Mehta. Narendra Mehta was born blind and developed an amazing sense of touch.He left his native India to study physical therapy in London. During his studies he was surprised that the Western physical therapy massage overlooked the importance of head massage and personalized aromatherapy (physiotherapists do not usually work with oils). He decided to get back to his roots and take pride in his ethnicity. He managed to combine what he was taught in India (Indian Head Massage is like a tradition that is passed on from generation to generation) with his knowledge of anatomy and physiotherapy.

Narendra Mehta is the author of the book *The Power of Touch*, and he and his wife are teachers dedicated to Indian Head and Face Massage. If you are ever in London, you can visit their Champissage Centre (Champi, or Champissage, is another name for Indian Head Massage).

"Incorporate Aromatherapy in your everyday living as a holistic treatment to promote overall well-being and healing on the physical, emotional and spiritual levels." - Deepak Chopra

Chapter 1: Understanding the Origins of Aromatherapy

The first evidence of the use of aromatherapy is believed to be the burning of tree gums, leaves, needles, and fragrant woods in ancient times. The beginning of this practice can be linked to the discovery that some woods used for making fire (such as cedar and cypress) filled the air with their scent when they burned.

It may sound surprising to you, but Aromatherapy, the term itself, was coined in the late 1920's, but in reality, for about hundreds and even thousands of years, roots of aromatic plants were used for making perfumes, incense and other medicinal purposes. Rather aromatic plants were used for medicinal and healing purposes way back in time as opposed to aromatic oils.

Some people may object when they hear that aromatherapy has been used for thousands of years. This is because they only associate aromatherapy withthe essential oils that are labeled and ready to use, something that our Western, scientific world is used to.

We usually tell them to trace some history; many ancient cultures were using aromatherapy daily for all kinds of rituals, they would also start developing their own aromatherapy and naturopathy for different ailments.

The Egyptians have been credited with the invention of the first distillation equipment around 3000 BC. It involved the infusion of rudimentary oils with herbs, the product of which was used in rituals, cosmetics, medicine, and perfumery. It was years later that Hippocrates (widely regarded as the "Father of Medicine") first studied how different essential oils had an effect in healing and for medicinal reasons, and hence promoted the use of these oils.

In India, the use of aromatic herbs can be traced through history, and was called *itr,* meaning 'fragrance' in Arabic. The history of *itr* is as old as the Indian civilization itself. The earliest instance of distillation of *itr* has been found in the Ayurvedic text called *Charaksamhita.* In 7th century AD, the *Harshacharita* mentions the use of fragrant agar wood oil.

Coming to the modern era, the field of aromatherapy was established as a field of science in an accidental discovery by Rene Maurice Gatttefosse, a French chemist, who, as we have already mentioned, is responsible for coining the term 'Aromatherapy'.

What happened is that Gatttefosse suffered from a burn injury while working in the lab. As a reflex, he dunked his hand in a tub of lavender oil, which was the nearest liquid. The burn healed quickly and without any scarring. This led him to research essential oils extensively. In 1937, Gatttefosse published the book titled *Aromathérapie: Les Huiles Essentielles Hormones Vegetales.*

This may be a little bit off topic now, but yesterday we had a family picnic in the local woods. We got back with several mosquito bites each. We applied one drop of lavender essential oil on each bite and both the swelling and the redness disappeared overnight. We are almost healed now! We also use bergamot oil as a mosquito repellent and on mosquito bites to stimulate healing. More on different modes of application in the following chapters!

While the original work was in French, later an English translation titled as *Aromatherapy* was published; this is in print even today.

Other famous Western Aroma Therapists are: Dr. Jean Valnetm who relied on Aromatherapy for treating WWII Soldiers, Madame Marguerite Maury, a biochemist from Austria who used aromatherapy in cosmetics and eventually for massage purposes, and Robert B Tisserand, who wrote the first book on Aromatherapy in English.

Though Aromatherapy is widely used across the world for healing and curing certain illnesses, in ancient times essential oils were used for mystical experiences. For example, frankincense has always been used for mystical meditation.

"Frankincense has, among its physical properties, the ability to slow down and deepen the breath...which is very conductive to prayer and meditation" (from Davis, P. London School of Aromatherapy notes)

Rosemary was used by Romans in religious or wedding ceremonies, in food and in cosmetics, and the Egyptians used it as incense. Since the study in Aromatherapy, Rosemary is now used for stimulating hair growth, boosting mental activity, reducing pain and relieving respiratory problems. As you can see, one essential oil is really multifunctional and can be used for treating a range of conditions.

In the same manner, thyme leaves that we find abundantly in the kitchen and our kitchen gardens is widely used in Aromatherapy. Thyme oil has been found useful in the treatment of digestive and respiratory conditions. So yes, there are many plant materials and herbs, which you use for cooking and other purposes that are vastly used in Aromatherapy.

The following chapters will help you discover some really refreshing, holistic self-care tips...

Chapter 2: Ayurvedic Aromatherapy as a Holistic Medicine

Unlike modern medicines, Ayurvedic Aromatherapy believes that a healthy body is the result of a perfect communion between the physical and spiritual self. It takes into consideration your everyday lifestyle and teaches you how to change your habits. The most extraordinarily striking part is that it gives your illness a chance to heal.

The underlying methodology behind all Ayurvedic treatments is a firm belief in the fact that prevention is better than cure. To a large extent that stands absolutely true in the case of most ailments. The focus therefore, is to prevent the germination of a disease rather than fretting later. Aromatherapy, therefore, can be seen as essential when people are struggling with stress issues and physical challenges almost on a daily basis.

Ayurvedic Aromatherapy uses essential oils to set into motion its larger objective of healing and recuperation, and it also ensures a healthy balance between a proper diet, exercise, herbs, meditation and yoga (of course, the focus on this book is on aromatherapy only). All this in turn leads to the treatment of a number of diseases and prevention of yet more in number.

Like we said earlier, Aromatherapy is an example of a perfect coupling of medication and nature. It goes back to nature and uses natural ingredients for treatment of various problems and deformities. Now, wouldn't you like to opt for natural treatments as opposed to modern day medicine to get relief from your illnesses?

It indeed is a growing challenge to the monopoly of the conventional medicines used over time as people are becoming more and more aware of Ayurveda and its therapeutic qualities and going the natural way. This is the reason that an entire tourism industry is booming in countries like India, Egypt and China, which specializes in natural oriental medicine. It's quite funny for us now, but one of our teachers used to say:

"I do not understand how come so many Westerners who are wealthy (from the authors: even if you think you are not rich, you will be considered rich when you go to countries like India) *and come from developed countries know less about proper*

self-care than my 7 year old son! How come they allowed so much negligence to take place and now they really need to get back to the roots!

I have also have students from Europe, North America and Australia who actually decided to stay in India and quit their jobs and break away from their Western social status. They were blown away by the quality of life that is achieved both thanks to how much money you are making, but also because WHO YOU BECOME and HOW YOU TAKE CARE OF YOURSELF AND THOSE AROUND YOU".

The commonly used ingredients in Ayurvedic Aromatherapy include herbs and oils extracted from numerous plants that have medicinal value. The oils extracted are supplied to the body in different ways, including adding them in bathing water, inhaling them, or using them in diluted form (essential oil diluted in good quality carrier cold-pressed oil).

If you are new to aromatherapy, and Ayurveda, let's have a look at some aromatherapy definitions that we will be using throughout this booklet:

Essential Oils (EO): these can be described as pure essences extracted from different parts of fruits, trees, flowers and stems. Even though they are called "oils", they are not oily at all.

Before employing essential oils topically, via massage, it is of paramount importance to first dilute them in good quality vegetable base oil (these are oily).

Test on a small area of skin first to make sure you are not allergic, because some people will break out in rashes/blister if it turns out they are allergic/sensitive to certain extracts. And that really takes the fun out of the whole experience.

The general rule of a thumb, that is typical of the English school of aromatherapy and one that we recommend to beginners, is to use up to 5 drops of your chosen essential oil, or oils, in one tablespoon of carrier oil (vegetable oil).

Ok, we understand that a tablespoon may differ on size sometimes, so let us tell you that by saying one tablespoon we mean about 15 ml.

Vegetable Oils (VO): These are the carrying oils. You will need them as a natural base for your massage treatments. They will be able to penetrate your skin and let the essential oils do their job.

Don't use poor quality mineral oils. Work only with natural vegetable oils.

Some Popular Ayurvedic Essential Oils (our favorites!):

- Lavender
- Bergamot
- Betel Leaf
- Black Cumin
- Black Pepper
- Birch
- Bakul Attar
- Rosewood
- Sambrani

Popular Ayurvedic Vegetable Oils:

- Sesame oil
- Jojoba oil
- Coconut oil
- Grape seed oil

32

Ayurvedic Aromatherapy does wonders in treating ailments as effectively as it fights stress and anxiety. This is the reason why more and more stressed out Westerners are turning towards it. It is a common practice these days to use Aromatherapy in close conjunction with massage therapy, phytotherapy and the likes.

The best part of Aromatherapy is that the treatment offered is personalized, because each person has a unique constitution, so in a way you will get a personalized Aromatherapy treatment based on your physical traits and needs.

Warm and energizing oils are used for people who are at a higher risk of headaches, hypersensitivity and insomnia. Sharp scents are avoided and warm scents are combined with calming oils. An amalgamation of oils extracted from camphor, cinnamon along with soothing ones like jasmine, rose and sandalwood are considered apt. This particular category of people falls under the *Vata* type (James).

The *Pitta* type of people who are prone to acidity, skin problems, inflammation, ulcers and fevers are easily agitated. They are treated by exposing them to cooling and soothing fragrances like sandalwood, rose and mint. For proper treatment, the carrier suited is coconut oil as opposed to sesame oil which is used as a carrier in case of the *Vata* people. The *Kapha* types who are predisposed to respiratory problems are said to benefit from light and warm oils like basil and cedar used with extremely light carrier oils. Sharp stimulating fragrances are also effective.

Ayurvedic Aromatherapy has made a tremendous contribution to the field of preventative care. It caters to a number of problems including acne, cold and flu, skin allergies, heart diseases and Alzheimer's disease. Herbs and essential oils provide prevention by building a stronger immune system. If you are harrowed by constant headaches or colds, then you should definitely opt for Aromatherapy treatments as a first line of defense.

It would not be wrong to categorize the technique as a holistic one that cares for everything. In fact, it is a great source of mental strength and goes a long way in providing a soothing effect on your mind.

There are a lot of stress-relieving oils that are used in Aromatherapy. These include:

- lavender,
- bergamot
- clary sage

Aromatherapy goes a long way in detoxifying the body, which is extremely important. Using Aromatherapy oils for bathing, massaging and rubbing the neck and abdomen has the potential for relieving the body of unnecessary toxins.

"By oil massage the human body becomes strong and smooth-skinned; it gains resistance to exhaustion and exertion"

Charak Samhita

AROMATHERAPY PRECAUTIONS

Aromatherapy General Precautions

Aromatherapy is a very safe and easy therapy to use, but keep in mind that there are certain precautions:

- Remember to wash your hands after applying aromatherapy massage;

- Do not apply the essential oils in their pure form as they may cause an allergic reaction. Instead, use blends that contain 2-5% essential oils diluted in good-quality cold-pressed oil;

-After using citrus oils, like for example lemon, verbena, bergamot, orange etc. avoid direct sun exposure, even up to 8 hours after the treatment

- Do not apply oils after surgery (unless you have consulted with a doctor) or on open wounds or rashes of unknown origin;

- Do not use the oils after chemotherapy (unless suggested by a doctor);

- Keep the oils away from the eyes and mucus membranes;

- Use the oils only topically (unless you have consulted with an aromatherapist who specializes in phytoaromatherapy);

- Avoid rosemary, thyme, Spanish and common sage, fennel and hyssop if you suffer from high blood pressure;

- Do not apply the treatments described in this book on babies or infants. It doesn't mean that aromatherapy can never be used on babies and infants, but extremely low concentrations should be used. Always consult with a medical or naturopathy doctor first;

- After an aromatherapy massage always remember to wash your hands;

- Make sure that you research the brand, read safety instructions for each individual oil you buy/use and check the expiration date;

- Store your blends in dark glass bottles, preferably in a cool, dry and dark place and remember to use within a maximum of one month after mixing.

Chapter 3: Mechanism and Mode of Application

Using aromatherapy is a real pleasure to the senses, it can offer an immediate relief for stressed out bodies and minds!

Vaporized odor molecules released by essential oils float in the air and then reach the nostrils, and quickly dissolve in the mucus, which is on the roof of each nostril.

The process may seem a little bit technical, but in reality it is pretty simple. The olfactory epithelium situated underneath the mucus paves way for the molecules to reach the olfactory receptors that are special receptors and the neurons detect the odor. The odor formed there is transferred to the olfactory bulbs situated at the back of the nose.

The olfactory bulbs are of primary importance. This is so because they are home to the sensory receptors, which actually form a pivotal part in the brain. The message catalyzed by the essential oils aim to cure the patient of a particular disease. It then gets transmitted to the brain centre, and these in turn have a substantial impact on emotions, memories and other higher levels of the consciousness.

In simple terms, the scent of certain oils and herbs has a soothing, calming effect and can cure certain illnesses. These herbs. when used in the right manner, can help build immunity and also help fight against many illnesses.

The mechanics behind Aromatherapy are still not completely understood and requires a lot more work to uncover its full potential. However, one thing you can be sure of, the aromas induced by the essential oils have an influence on the brain and an impact on the **limbic structure** (it is responsible for pleasant feelings and emotions) this can help you in keeping many conditions at bay, without the help of any synthetic drugs or medication.

There is also more to it- imagine that you get back home from work after a really stressful day. You treat yourself to a nice aromatherapy bath and then you massage your body with your chosen vegetable oil with a few drops of your chosen Ayurvedic essential oil, or oils. What will happen is that the oils will penetrate your skin and will finally get absorbed to your circulatory system. They will then continue their healing job of detoxifying and stimulating your immune system.

Of course, during the aromatherapy massage (both self-massage and one you can get from the hands of an experienced Ayurvedic masseuse), you will also experience the pleasure of aromas, as we have previously discussed. So, to sum up, it's like 2 in 1 treatment. The effect on your olfactory tract and the limbic system of the brain is almost immediate while when applied on the skin, it may take a few hours to penetrate your system and do the healing. This is why, after aromatherapy massage, we recommend you do not shower for about 8 hours. We are both in habit of doing our personalized aromatherapy massages before we go to sleep.

We don't use any body lotions or milks (unless they are organic), we only use natural oils that we know work for us. We don't like lots of different products accumulating on our bathroom shelves, we prefer just a couple of cold pressed vegetable oils that we use as a base for our treatments and a range of essential oils that we mix and blend with the vegetable oils to personalize our treatments.

The reason is simple- we don't want any artificial ingredients on our body. You may be wondering: "does it mean I can't use any creams or lotions"?

The answer is- you can use them as long as they are pure and organic.

Natural lotions and creams are great as a base for aromatherapy treatments.

We normally use vegetable oils or aloe vera gel though. We just got used to using them on a regular basis and we find them multifunctional.

Different Modes of Application

Ayurvedic Aromatherapy is quite diverse in its application and therefore can be made available through a number of means, depending upon your needs, time, work and requirements. The three widely accepted modes of application are topical application (we have already mentioned massage and self-massage Abhyanga treatments), direct inhalation and aerial diffusion.

1. Aerial diffusion is similar to environmental fragrance. Its purpose is to fill a room with a natural fragrance. You could make use of certain simple methods and devices to carry out the diffusion effectively. Simple tissue diffusion is easy, convenient and easily transferable.

It is very instrumental in a workplace or a public place as you could easily complete it by putting drops of aroma on a tissue and the aroma itself diffuses as you move around.

Steam diffusion however, is a faster means of diffusing an aroma in a room. The steam helps to heat the oil and thereby bring about a faster diffusion of oils in the air. Candle diffusion also works for a lot of people, and hence you see a lot of variety of aromatherapy candles in stores and wellness clinics. However, the essential oils are generally flammable, so this method demands a lot of caution (essential oils need to be kept away from the direct flame). The aroma is not long-lasting and sometimes, due to the heat, its effect might fade away faster. Yes, but if you are just looking for relaxing your senses, then candles may do the trick.

There are many commercial products available these days that can help in diffusion. These include lamp ring diffusers made of terracotta or brass. The best part about them is they are not expensive; rather they are efficient to carry out a desired purpose. Fan diffusers are also available in the market, and they help to diffuse the aroma in the air. Electric heat diffusers are effective in spreading the fragrance in a larger area and are also more productive when it comes to thicker oils. Oil nebulizers can also be considered as one of the many options available in the market. This is an excellent way to create a nice atmosphere in your house and improve your well-being in only a few seconds.

2. Direct inhalation is a means of disinfecting the respiratory system. It helps decrease congestion, increases and enables expectoration and also psychologically enhances your moods and energies. Among the many advantages of direct inhalation are stimulation of the brain and immune system, mood enhancement and relaxation.

In this method, you breathe the evaporating oil straight in. It could be done easily by placing a few drops of your chosen essential oil on the wrists and rubbing them together. The hands should then be cupped over the face carefully protecting the eyes and thereafter the oil should be inhaled three to five times.

One could also inhale directly from the bottle- just open it and take a few deep aroma breaths. I, Elena, always carry bergamot essential oil in my bag as it helps me relax and think clearly. I am very often exposed to stress because of work and my business. Aromatherapy is soothing for me and imparts a calming effect on my body, mind and emotions. I never let the tension accumulate; I prevent it from taking over my body. I know that thanks to aromatherapy self-care that I do on a regular basis, I am more successful and productive at work, with my clients and enjoying time with my family.

James finds relief in oils like clove or basil. We both think that they have mysterious, masculine scent.

Inhalation is sometimes preferred over other methods, especially in cases where the goal is weight loss, growth hormone secretion or even balancing emotions.

We are not saying that aromatherapy is like a weight loss cure, but it is a great complimentary therapy to help you prevent overeating and can help you change your relationship with food.

3. Topical application is manifested in baths, massages, compresses and the likes. These in fact form the backbone of the popular perception of Ayurvedic Aromatherapy. Very commonly employed, these means are popularized a great deal by the spa centers and the emerging tourism and hospitality industry. The means employed in topical application are said to ensure and facilitate a healthy blood circulation, pain relief and thereby restoring a stress-free life.

- Hot compresses are no less than a blessing for people susceptible to migraine headaches, sore muscles and sinus headaches. Peppermint oils, rosewood and neroli are recommended in this case. You can follow these remedies from the comforts of your home and see the effect for yourself.

45

- It follows a simple method to soak a piece of clothing in hot water, which has drops of the essential oil added, and place the cloth on the patient's head, repeating the process. Instant relief is guaranteed.

- A hot bath will not only provide you relaxation but it will also relieve the mucus and replenish your skin. It's not only about relaxation, it can also help you heal skin allergies and improve lymph circulation.

Lemon, cedar wood and rosemary are the perfect, and most commonly used, essential oils employed in massages. They are a great source of getting rid of tension and relieving pain and stress. Massages are the most commonly employed means of spreading the spark of Ayurvedic Aromatherapy. Carrier lotions or oils (called base oils or vegetable oils as mentioned in the previous chapter) assume importance in this case. The most commonly used lotions are almond, Shea and cocoa butter blended with the essential oils to suit the purpose.

You may notice that a lot of the natural and organic lotions and creams that you may be using contain the above aromatic ingredients. These have physical and psychological benefits that can be experienced after a soothing bath. The olfactory senses are triggered and some oils even have the potential to blend in the skin and impart medicinal values by healing the skin of a particular problem.

There are a variety of oils to choose from with different values and a distinct flavor to them. For example, peppermint has exceptional energizing values and lavender is said to be more of a soothing agent. In some cases, lavender is even considered safe without dilution. Do you remember our encounter with mosquitoes in the local woods? We applied a drop of lavender oil on each mosquito bite. Cold packs of essential oils can be used to cure swollen tissues.

Topical application would be more effective if the oils are used in a way to make them stay in longer contact with the skin. The more effectively they are absorbed, more effective they would be in healing. The evaporation of the oils can be prevented by keeping them under a layer of synthetic-free lotion. This enhances penetration. Muscle injuries or injuries in bones and ligaments are more effectively dealt with topical application. The topical method application also works quite well with acupressure.

Back to your base oils, always make sure that they are not minerals oils and are synthetic free. The reason for that is simple; the chemical ingredients create a chemical layer on your skin and prevent the healing essential oils from penetrating it. Such a treatment may of course give you some nice and pleasant aromas for a few seconds or minutes but is really far away from out holistic Ayurvedic aromatherapy.

These three are therefore only different methods to make full use of the bounties of Ayurvedic Aromatherapy. You could easily make a choice and pick the methodology of application best suited to the situation at hand and reap the benefits of Aromatherapy.

Chapter 4: Aromatherapy-Methods

Like other medicinal divisions, Aromatherapy applies its own ingredients and materials that help in the curing process. Some of the common materials employed for practicing and treating with Aromatherapy are as follows:

Essential Oils

We already discussed that essential oils first came into the commercial picture in 1920's, when Rene Maurice Gatttefosse, a French chemist had burned his hand in a laboratory explosion; he used lavender oil. Its antiseptic properties, which delineated from chemical ones, were quite helpful to heal his hand. This drew his attention towards the dermatological aspect of lavender oil and consequently other oils, too. While working in his family's perfume company, he became interested in the antiseptic value of these oils. Eventually, he coined the term *Aromatherepie* and published a book with the same name by 1937.

Later, other French doctors like Jean Valet would use these essential oils in the treatment of soldiers and sometimes to treat psychiatric patients despite much skepticism by other doctors. He continued the work of Gatttefosse in *Aromathérapie*.

Essential oils, compared against their chemical counterparts. are seen to be more responsive and subtle, due to multiple properties that oil constitutes within itself. Chemical ones on the contrary carry within them usually a single property where their sole aim is to fix the problem since they are tailored to do so.

Essential oils have a balancing effect; their sole motive is more than treating a specific problem. It takes the idea of balancing from Ayurveda, which follow the principle of balancing.

These same qualities are followed in case of psychological imbalances such as depression, mood swings, hysteria. For long these have been considered as an excess of one of the humors. Considering this imbalanced state, these essential oils cater to your well being through their fragrance that gives a therapeutic effect to your mind. These are seen as better alternatives than conventional psychotropic drugs. Moreover, human contact while massaging, forms an important extension of Aromatherapy.

It is always advised to use prescribed essential oils and use them in right amounts by consulting an Aroma therapist, since insufficient knowledge can lead to hazardous results. What we offer in this book are simple self-treatments to be performed at home, but if you are on medication or suffer from any serious condition, or are pregnant, we strongly recommend you consult your local Ayurvedic or aromatherapy practitioner first.

Absolutes

As opposed to essential oils, which require steam distillation for preparation, absolutes on the contrary use the method of solvent extraction and enfluerage - a process that uses solid, odorless fats at room temperature in order to capture the fragrance of the plant. These processes are used especially in case of flower petals where there is lesser risk of breaking, unlike distillation.

The process of enfluerage yields a material known as '*pomade*', which is a mixture of essential oils and fats, while that of solvent extraction produces a concrete of waxes, fats, essential oils and other plant materials. This pomade and concrete is treated with alcohol in order to extract the absolute.

This absolute which is produced is essentially a highly concentrated, highly-aromatic, oily mixture. This process is usually run at low temperatures so as to avoid breakage of these petals. Since these have high aromatic and therapeutic effects, even a slight concentration of this absolute becomes sufficient. In case of rose absolutes, they solidify when kept at room temperatures, however when they are held in the hand these liquefy.

Often, the usage of absolutes is avoided since it carries with itself a few traces of solvents, even after extraction from the concrete or *pomade*. These can be harmful; however sometimes these are used by Aroma therapists in low quantities.

Carrier Oils

Commonly known as vegetable oils or base oils, carrier oils are used for diluting essential oils and absolute oils for topical application for massages and in Aromatherapy. They absorb the essential oils into the skin. Unlike essential oils, they don't contain any sort of concentrated aroma; however, some oils like olive oil have a mild smell.

These do not evaporate like essential oils, which are volatile. The carrier oils used should be as natural and unadulterated as possible. Cold-pressing and maceration are the two main methods of producing carrier oils. These methods are as follows:

Cold pressed method: In this process you need to make sure that the therapeutic acids and vitamins do not get destroyed. You need to avoid excessive heat for minimizing the changes in the innate properties of the oils.

Maceration: These carrier oils have added properties with respect to its production. In this method, parts of particular plants are cut and mixed with certain carrier oils like olive oil or sunflower oil. This mix is gently stirred for a certain span of time and then stored in a warm area. All the essential oils are then transferred in to the carrier oil and then the macerated mix is carefully filtered, so that the excess plant material can be separated.

You must have noticed that oils used for culinary purposes are often used for massages, which are again economical. Considering the presence of a range of different carrier oils each with various therapeutic properties, the choice of appropriate oil will depend on the area that will be massaged, skin sensitivity and the individual's requirements. Viscosity is a major consideration; for instance, grape seed oil is very thin, while olive oil is much thicker. Sunflower and sweet almond have a viscosity in between.

Infusions

The process of removing the flavors or chemical compounds from the plants in to a solvent like water, alcohol or some sort of oil is called infusion. In this method, it is required to allow the plant material to stay suspended inside the solvent for some time. The resultant liquid is called as the infusion.

The plant materials are used as dry herbs, berries or flowers. The liquid (oil, water or alcohol) is boiled to the right temperature and then dispensed on the herb. The liquid is either strained to remove the plants, or the herbs are separated from the liquid. The infusion is then refrigerated or bottled for later use.

Phytoncides

Phytoncides are antimicrobial chemical compounds that are derived from plants. Coined by Russian Biochemist, Dr. Boris P Tokin, Phytoncides literally mean, "something that is exterminated from the plant". As per Dr. Tokin, certain plants excrete active ingredients that prevent them from being eaten by insects and from rotting.

Some good examples of Phytoncides are spice, garlic, onion, oak tree, tea tree and pine tree. These substances defend the plants from bacterial and fungal growth.

Chapter 5: Popular Oils

Aromatherapy employs a lot of different fragrant oils that have healing and soothing properties. You will notice that most of them are made from commonly used herbs and flowers. Let's dive into it!

Thyme Oil

Thyme oil is reddish-brown to amber in color and has a sweet and strong herbal smell. It is extracted from steam or distillation of the fresh/partly dried flowering tops and leaves of the thyme plant. It was used in ancient times by the Greeks, the Romans, and the Egyptians for medicinal purposes.

The oil derives its name from the Greek word 'thymos' which means 'perfume' which is related to its use as incense in Greek temples. The Egyptians also used it in the embalming process.

Thyme oil is found to strengthen the nerves and enhance concentration and memory. It is also recommended as a natural remedy for the following conditions:

- Depression
- Colds
- Catarrh
- Sinusitis
- Sore throat
- Tonsillitis

Thyme has a warming effect on the area of application and is also helpful in treating:
- Poor circulation
- Muscular aches
- Sprains
- Obesity and edema
- Irregular periods
- Cellulite

It is a natural antiseptic; we always use it in winter to prevent colds and flu.

Thyme oil blends particularly well with lemon, grapefruit, bergamot, rosemary, pine and lavender.

Peppermint Oil

A native to the Mediterranean, the pale yellow peppermint oil has a fresh and sharp, menthol-like smell. It is extracted from a perennial herb that has slight, saw-like leaves and pink/mauve flowers. It is extracted using the steam distillation method from the body of the plant (either fresh or partly dried) that is on the surface of the ground before flowering.

This herb has many species and this might produce varieties of the oil with slight differences. Peppermint piperita is a hybrid of two such sub-species, spearmint (M. spicata) and watermint (M. aquatica).

Peppermint oil is excellent for several skin related problems like skin irritation, itchiness, skin redness due to inflammation (in which case the cooling effect of the oil on skin helps). It is used for acne, dermatitis, scabies, ringworm and pruritus, and also for relieving itching or sunburn.

Peppermint oil provides the natural cure for a range of problems related to the digestive system for example:

- Cramps
- Nausea
- Colic
- flatuence

It also helps in relieving pain in cases of:
- toothache,
- neuralgia,
- rheumatism,
- menstrual cramps,
- foot ache and other muscular pains.

The effect of peppermint oil on the mind is observed in its ability to refresh the spirit and stimulate mental agility. It relieves the mind of fatigue and depression and also improves concentration.

I, James, always have some peppermint essential oil in my office. When I feel like I get stuck with a project, I use it with my diffuser, or sometimes I take a 15 minute break for a mini self-massage. I mix 2 drops of peppermint oil with a teaspoon of coconut oil and I massage my neck and my ears. It helps me refresh and very often calm down my vita-pita tendencies.

Benzoin, lemon, rosemary, lavender, marjoram and eucalyptus are some of the oils that blend well with peppermint oil.

Elena really enjoys blending peppermint oil with cinnamon oil- we both think it's a greatly stimulating aphrodisiac and we recommend you try it with your partner.

Peppermint also makes an amazing blend with citric scents, like for example bergamot, verbena, lemon, or sweet orange. We find such blends suitable for both if us, even though we are different doshas. While a peppermint scent is cooling and refreshing (perfect for people with pitta tendencies who get angry and red easily!), citrus scents are slightly uplifting (great for kaphas who have tendency to get stuck or even lazy). Of course, we are making it really general now, but we hope you get the way it works. We also encourage you to try aromatherapy and work on balancing your dosha, and most importantly, understanding practicing and feeling it

Lavandula Oil

An extract of Lavandula Augustifolia, Lavandula oil is more popularly known as lavender oil. This oil has a clear color along with watery viscosity. It has a fresh aroma and has been used in bath routines since the ancient times among the Romans.

Lavandula oil has a very soothing effect. It revitalizes and tones different types of skin issues like oily skin, acne, burns, boils, insect bites, lice, and stings.

You can use it as mosquito repellant. It also has the capacity to relax the nerves, to relieve tension, panic, depression, hysteria, migraines, headaches and insomnia.

It helps with several ailments related to the digestive system (vomiting, nausea, colic and flatulence) and the respiratory system (asthma, colds, throat infections, halitosis, whooping coughs, laryngitis and bronchitis).

Lavandula oil is also beneficial in relieving pain in cases of arthritis, rheumatism, lumbago and muscular pains, especially those related to sporting activities.

Lavender oil particularly blends well with other oils like pine, geranium, all kinds of citrus oils, clary sage and cedar wood.

Jasmine Oil

Jasmine essential oil has a sweet and floral smell. It is extracted from the white-star shaped flowers of the jasmine shrubs which are evergreen, fragile creepers that can grow up to 10 meters. It is picked at night when its aroma is at its peak. Jasmine oil has been used for medicinal purposes since the ancient times by the Chinese, Indians and the Arabians. It was also used as an aphrodisiac as well as for other ceremonial purposes.

Because of its soothing floral smell, it produces a feeling of euphoria, confidence and optimism. It soothes the nerves, overcomes the feelings of depression and revitalizes and restores energy. Again because of its deeply calming nature, jasmine oil helps with a number of sexual problems such as premature ejaculation, impotency and frigidity (hence, its ancient use is as of aphrodisiac).

This oil is non-toxic, non-irritant and generally also non-sensitizing. Thus, it does not show any side-effects. However, some people might have an allergic reaction to jasmine oil. The therapeutic properties of jasmine oil which determines its various applications are aphrodisiac, antiseptic, anti-depressant, anti-spasmodic, expectorant, cicatrisant, parturient, galactagogue, uterine and sedative.

Jasmine oil is a great natural remedy for sensitive and greasy complexions. Aside from facial treatments, ayurvedic spas use it to reduce stretch marks.

Jasmine oil has a very beneficial effect on ailments related to the respiratory system. It soothes irritating coughs and helps with laryngitis and hoarseness.

The essential oils that Jasmine oil blends particularly well with are rose, bergamot, sandalwood and all citrus oils.

Chapter 6: Using Ayurvedic Aromatherapy for Common Ailments

Oils used in Aromatherapy can be absorbed through the pores in your skin or through the nose. Oils are easily sensed by the receptors in your nose, which carry it to the brain with the help of neurons. Often the oils are applied to the palms of the hand or the bottom of the feet from where they are absorbed into the blood stream in less than five minutes.

<u>Acne</u>

There is an array of essential oils that can help you control and prevent the problem of acne. Aromatherapy not just clears the skin but does it by helping the management of the very underlying problems that cause acne. They regulate the oil production by the oil glands under the skin, balance hormones and regulate fluctuations, reduce stress, and improve the complexion.

This is why Aromatherapy is the ideal treatment for your acne problems like pimples, blemishes, and other types of skin eruptions. This is the reason why even chemical products in the market claim to have been inspired by an Ayurvedic formula containing essential oils such as eucalyptus oil, lemon or lavender. Essential oils are also effective in fighting off bacteria from the acne affected region.

The best essential oils for acne treatment are:
- eucalyptus
- geranium
- wood
- sandalwood
- lemongrass
- frankincense
- lavender
- tree
- clary sage
- juniper berry
- lemon
- bergamot
- verbena

Base oils recommended for anti-acne treatments are hazelnut oil, coconut oil as well as aloe vera gel (this one has a really nice, light consistency and is perfect for hot summers).

Addiction

Lately, Aromatherapy has become a popular therapeutic practice in treating the withdrawal symptoms during a drug addiction treatment. Though varying according to the addiction of drug, withdrawal symptoms generally include sleep disturbances, restlessness, irritability and anxiety. Essential oils used in Aromatherapy help to create an emotional balance, promoting a sense of calm by reducing the feelings of stress. The result of this is a considerable reduction in several withdrawal symptoms.

Aromatherapy is mostly used as an adjunct to support the traditional addiction treatment methods. Aromatherapy, when combined with massage therapy, considerably improves the therapeutic value of the latter. It produces a greater sense of holistic well-being because of an increased sense of relaxation and healing of pain.

Below listed are some of the Aromatherapy essential oils that are especially beneficial in treatment of withdrawal symptoms:

- **Anise Aromatherapy:** Anise curbs cravings for chocolate or sugary items, which are often experienced by those fighting alcohol addictions. It also relieves stress and induces better sleep and provides relaxation.

- **Chamomile Aromatherapy:** Chamomile has been traditionally regarded as an antidepressant. It helps to relieve suppressed anger, and thus provides relaxation and aids sleep. Helpful in fighting cravings and addictions

- **Frankincense Aromatherapy:** Frankincense induces spirituality, clears perception, and leads to higher states of consciousness. It encourages a kind of optimism and also helps in a release from the past. It is also effective in combating cravings for sugar or sedatives.

- **Lavender Aromatherapy:** Lavender provides relief from lethargy and exhaustion due to work, calms the nerves, thus helping during the withdrawal phase. It also reduces cravings for alcohol.

- **Fennel Aromatherapy:** Fennel also helps in dispelling cravings for chocolate, alcohol and sugar, common during the withdrawal phase.

Alzheimer's disease and other forms of dementia

Yes, it may sound quite surprising but it is true, Aromatherapy plays an important role in treating dementia and Alzheimer's disease to a great extent. People suffering from Alzheimer's disease or other forms of dementia frequently experience states of agitation that makes them a challenge to their family or caregivers.

Traditional medication involves the use of strong tranquilizers that suppress such feelings of agitation, but it is generally accompanied by partial or full unconsciousness of the patient. Thus, Ayurvedic Aromatherapy becomes an important form of alternative medication in which essential oils are applied to the patients through methods like massage, direct inhalation, bath, ambient diffusion etc.

Different essential oils show varying properties. Some popular and easily available essential oils used in the medication of dementia include:

- **Lavender**: It is an antidepressant which calms the nerves and balances strong emotions. It is also good for insomnia, thus, promoting better sleep and a better overall mood.

- **Rosemary**: Rosemary essential oil stimulates body and mind, creating a feeling of emotional well being. It also improves the cognitive performance of the mind in its accuracy and also in terms of speed.

- **Peppermint:** When used in the morning, it boosts appetite. It stimulates the mind and calms the nerves. It is also helpful in keeping a check on absent-mindedness caused by dementia.

- **Lemon Balm**: It induces a feeling of calmness and relaxation and is very effective in cases of anxiety and insomnia.

Chapter 7: Ayurvedic Spa at Home

In order to select an essential oil, an Aroma therapist carefully studies the patient, which includes his lifestyle, eating pattern, emotional and behavioral pattern. This is known as a holistic examination in Aromatherapy. Keeping this approach in mind, in correspondence to *doshas*, various essential oils are recommended.

We encourage you to be your own patient.

We have included a <u>bonus chapter</u>. We recommend you have a look at our mini dosha test.

We think that discovering your prevalent dosha is really exciting; it's like getting to know yourself. You can also do the test with your family and friends.

These are just the general examples as for some oils that your dosha may like:

- ***Vata*** **likes** ginger, cinnamon, camphor, rosewood, anise, angelica, lemon, eucalyptus and basil

- **_Pitta likes_** chamomile, yarrow, lime, coriander, sandalwood, and peppermint.

- **_Kapha likes_** sage, rosemary, naiouli, and clove

Considering the three basic body types, it is necessary to know the 'imbalance' caused due to excess of any of the _doshas_.

For example, if you experience anger, ulcers and agitation, you should try to balance pitta, and therefore should choose oils that pita dosha likes (calming and relaxing).

Vata

- Symptoms: In this, you are susceptible to headaches, nervous anxiety, hypersensitivity, dry skin, and constipation.
- Precautions: Avoid sharp-perfumed essential oils.
- Sources: Warm and stimulating oils like camphor, cypress and cinnamon, along with calming and stabilizing oils like jasmine, rose, sandalwood are blended in sesame oil, as it has the ability to penetrate in to the skin.

Pitta

- Symptoms: Ulcers, acidity, fevers, agitation, inflammatory skin diseases and anger
- Sources: Oils that give a cooling effect usually with fragrances of flowers like jasmine, gardenia, rose, mint and sandalwood, which are blended in to a cooling carrier oil like coconut oil.

Kapha

- Symptoms: Respiratory ailments

- Sources: Oils that have a warm effect like basil, cedar, pine and sage. Sharp fragrances that have a stimulating effect can also be beneficial.

AYURVEDIC SPA TIPS FOR VATA:

Self-Massage (self- Abhy, or: Abhyanga) for vattas that need more focus, balance and warmth to balance their dosha.

You can get back on track, relax, rejuvenate and detoxify with the following oils that we recommend:

VEGETABLE BASE OILS:

- Coconut oil
- Jojoba oil
- Almond oil
- Safflower oil
- Sesame Oil

ESSENTIAL OILS:

- Basil (James loves it, we have mentioned it before, haven't we?)
- Patchouli
- Vetiver

The proportion for a full body massage is more or less:

2 tablespoons of your chosen vegetable oil + about 10 drops (in total) of your chosen essential oil (or oils if you blend more than 1).

If you are new to aromatherapy or to particular oils, we suggest you test your blend on a small area of skin, for example on your forearm.

Now, since James is quite tall and athletic and he does not shave his legs or chest, he needs more oils (about 3 tablespoons + 15 drops of essential oils).

Elena, on the other hand is small and thin. She does shave her legs, haha and does not have any hair on her chest yet this is why she can do with small amount of oils, like for example: 1 tablespoon + 5 drops of her chosen essential oils (she loves 2 drops of bergamot + 3 drops of mint, great for her kapha nature.

Additionally, we recommend you use stones for self-massage. It's very easy, just press the points on your body where the tension is. For example, James tends to accumulate tension in his neck. This happens after long hours of writing as well as emotional stress that he may sometimes fall victim of. If you are vatta, simply touch and press the affected areas with one or more of the following stones:

- Tiger eye
- Lapis Lazuli (also for pitas, great for insomnia and restlessness, if you are a workaholic, you have just found your stone)
- Emerald
- Cat's eye
- Amethyst

You can also sleep with them. Yes! Put them under the pillow or on your night table. You can also meditate with them, carry them in your bad or keep them in your office. Wash them regularly with cold water and sea salt so as to purify their energy field. They will heal and balance your chakras and result in your ultimate wellness!

Vatta people, like for example James, are very creative. They put their heart and soul into their work. This is why they very often feel burnt out and as a result experience lack of energy and even anxiousness and nervousness.

This is why we recommend you get some highly therapeutic ayurvedic herbs and infusions and use them in your health spa. Don't drink coffee nor back tea. It will only aggravate your condition. There is a range of vata friendly and balancing drinks:

- cinnamon bark,
- chicory root, organic
- ginger root,
- cardamom,
- nutmeg
- mint
- chamomile

You can use them separately or mix them.

James likes to relax in a nice, warm bath with aromatherapy (he likes basil, as you already know, but he also likes sweet calming and grounding scents like: rose, angelica, bergamot (Elena loves it too), chamomile and vanilla.

We also both think that ylang ylang is a great idea for a nice and warm bath for two! It is an aphrodisiac, so be careful!

Simply add a few drops of your chosen essential oil or oils to your bath when the water is not running. Remember to stir the water energetically before you jump in- you want to make sure that essential oils are equally distributed.

So, while relaxing in his bath, James likes to enjoy his ayrvedic herbs and herbal teas. Before discovering Ayurveda, James used to resort to alcohol and drugs (bad idea!) and these would only aggravate his vata condition (he has pitta tendencies also which means that he can hit the roof easily).

Does he want to go back to where he was before?

No, because ayurvedic sensation of "feeling good" is just awesome!

AYURVEDIC SPA TIPS FOR KAPHA:

If you are kapha, you may need some holistic treatments to get your inspiration back and put you back on track. No slacking off!

Now you know the procedure of self-massage. If you are kapha, like Elena (if you are still unsure, check out the BONUS chapter, and follow our dosha test, it's fun!) your body and mind will be grateful for a regular self-massage with one or more of the following oils (you already know that essential oils must be first diluted in a vegetable base oil, so let's get straight to the point!).

Vegetable Oils:

- coconut oil
- mustard seed (really energizing) oil
- almond oil
- grape seed oil

(Elena recommends it for facial treatments, it is a natural anti-wrinkle treatment)

Essential Oils:

- Bergamot
- Lemon
- Pepper Mint
- Juniper
- Fennel
- Allspice
- Cinnamon
- Clove
- Lime
- Marjoram
- Thyme
- Myrrh
- Myrtle

Additional Therapies

Stones for self-massage, meditation and balancing for kapha people:

- Coral
- Sunstone
- Red Jasper
- Garnet

Herbs that we recommend if you tend to have kapha properties (lack of motivation, laziness, lack of productive energy, overeating, weight gain, oversleeping, and toxin accumulation- what a marvelous combination! Luckily, we know how to get to the root of the problem with ayurvedic aromatherapy and ayurvedic herbal infusions):

- Allspice
- Black pepper
- Rosemary
- Cinammon
- Coriander
- Turmeric

In short, we want something spicy, sexy and invigorating. This is what kaphas need.

Now, you may be tempted to drink coffe. You are probably thinking: "hey, if I am Kapha I need to wake up. Where is my mega cup of morning coffee?".

This is what we used to think as well, and if you ask Elena, she used to be a coffee addict...Unfortunately, what goes up must go down (even faster). Around midday Elena would suffer from horrible headaches and migraines. She would feel even more tired. This is why she finally learned how to listen to her amazing body and give it what it needs- natural, herbal stimulation that was designed for her dosha by the Mother Nature!

Kapha people tend to suffer from slow metabolism and usually have it difficult to lose weight. Include the mix of herbal infusions that we suggested and you will be amazed at the results.

If you suffer from toxin accumulation, fat accumulation and water retention, then do your daily Abhyanga and create your internal pharmacy with the following essential oils:

- Grapefruit
- Peppermint
- Juniper
- Fennel

You should focus on your stomach area.

The blend that Elena loves is the following:

- 1 tablespoon of coconutoil
- 4 drops of rosemary essential oil
- 2 drops of pepper mint essential oil
- 2 drops of lemon essential oil
- 2 drops of grapefruit essential oil
- 1 drop of frankincense essential oil

Apply on your belly and legs. Use energetic frictions and rub the area. You want to go as red as you can to stimulate your internal detoxifying energy that has been dormant for years!

If you suffer from constipation, massage your stomach and lumbar area with the following mix (perform 3 times a day, 2 hours after your meal):

- 1 tablespoon of your chosen vegetable oil
- 2 drops of peppermint oil
- 2 drops of clove
- 2 drops of allspice
- 2 drops of sweet orange oil

AYURVEDIC SPA TIPS FOR PITTA

The biggest obstacle that pitta people are facing is to keep calm, don't get that revved up, and to be patient. Things can sort themselves out naturally, there is no need to be such a control freak and have everyone do what you say.

We hope that you get this comparison! Pitta people have also tendency to work too much. While ayurveda is not the ultimate workaholism cure and much more work is needed on the mental level, ayurvedic aromatherapy and other natural therapies can soothe pitas and give them some well-deserved rest.

Like we said, pitas are always on fire. When under stress, they tend to work even harder. One of our best friends, John, is the most "pitta-like" person we have ever met. Everything in him is pitta, both his looks and his character. Not long ago, he was going through a painful divorce and he felt depressed. Now, here is a big difference between people that are kapha and people that are pitta. Kapha people, when depressed, tend to stay in and lead a life as a recluse. Pittas, on the other hand, get suckered into a whirl of work and intense partying and socializing. Both of these patterns are unbalancing and destroying.

Luckily, John is now recovered and back on track. In fact, he started dating again. His new girlfriend is also pitta and they are now both learning how to balance their explosive natures. They want their relationship to last, and two pitas on fire are a great match for a Latin telenovela, but not for a peaceful and balanced relationship that both John and his new partner seek...

People like John need calming, soothing and rejuvenating ayurvedic spa daily.

The tips that our friend is following now, include, of course the following ayurvedic natural therapies:

Self-Massage (do you remember how it is called in Ayurveda...? If you don't, then you have something of an absent-minded vata quality in you...!)

Vegetable Oils:

- Coconut oil (this one is the most famous one, come on, everyone loves coconut oil, it's like a living legend!)
- Sunflower
- Olive
- Almond

Essential Oils:

- Lavender
- Lavandin
- Chamomile
- Geranium
- Lemongrass
- Yatamansi
- Sandalwood (this one is really popular at ayurvedic health spas)

Stones:

- Lapis
- Yade
- Perdiot
- Pearl

- Emerald

Anger is an energy vampire. The more you hit the roof, the more tired you will feel. We suggest you try to cool down and chill out with the following herbal infusions:

- Spearmint
- Corriander

They seem to be working perfectly for John!

Now, it wasn't easy to convince John to get started on ayurveda. You see, typical pitas are really stubborn and set in their ways. They also tend to overindulge in foods that are not necessarily good for them (can be also alcohol, drugs and smoking- bad combination!). This is why they easily inflammable nature and very often bad habits result in digestive problems (acidity, ulcers). If this is something you are prone to, take action with your ayurvedic spa. Drink your soothing infusions daily and treat yourself to an aromatic massage. You can also ask your partner. John and his new girlfriend got really hooked on aromatherapy now! It's also a great time to develop intimacy with your partner. So much better than just watching TV (We don't recommend it, unless you want to kill your sex life forever!).

Here are some super soothing and relaxing blends for full-body massage for pitas.

Chill out Pitta Blend dedicated to our inspiring friend, John:

- 2 tablespoons of coconut oil
- 3 drops of Sandalwoodessential oil
- 5 drops of Lavender essential oil
- 3 drops of Chamomile essential oil

Apply as a full body massage.

If you feel like on the verge of hitting the roof, massage your face, forehead and scalp with the following blend:

- 1 tablespoon of your chosen vegetable oil
- 2 drops of peppermint essential oil
- 2 drops of geranium essential oil
- 2 drops of coriander essential oil

Massage gently for about 15 minutes. Breathe in and out. Leave in for about an hour. This is also a fantastic treatment to make your hair follicles stronger and so your hair- healthier.

This brings us to another healthy ayurvedic spa ritual.

Let's get started on our HOLISTIC HAIR SPA inspired by Ayurvedic Head Massage!

We both think that nowadays people use too many chemical shampoos and too many conditioners. It's both expensive and unhealthy. Back in India we did training in Indian Head Massage and we fell in love with this therapy. We will surely write a book on ayurvedic self-massage techniques, but for now we will only focus on aromatherapy that you can use both to improve your hair condition and to achieve deep, **holistic state of relaxation.**

We do this treatment at least twice a week.

The rules are very simple: before you wash your hair, apply your chosen oils on your scalp and massage energetically. Try to move the scalp as much as possible; the oils are full of nutrients that are excellent for hair follicles. They also penetrate and nourish the hair and can even treat the split ends.

You can either do this treatment 1 hour before washing your hair (it's good to massage your head for at least 15 minutes and then keep the oils for at least half an hour) or you can do it at nighttime and wash your hair the following day. We really recommend this treatment for damaged hair.

How to blend the oils?

We recommend that you use about 2 tablespoons of your chosen vegetable oil and up to 20 drops of your chosen essential oil, or oils if you are blending more than 1.

Vegetable oils for head massage

Choose your vegetable oil according to your dosha. We really love: coconut oil, sesame Oil and sweet almond oil.

Then, personalize your blend using essential oils depending on your hair type and possible conditions you want to eliminate.

You can also add a few drops of your chosen essential oil to your organic shampoo or, if you are using one, to your organic conditioner. The effect will be spectacular- super strong, healthy and shiny hair!

OILY HAIR-chamomile, grapefruit, lemongrass, lemon

DRY HAIR-ylang ylang, rosewood, sandalwood, palmarosa

STIMULATE HAIR GROWTH-rosemary, juniper, grapefruit

FIGHT DANDRUFF AND ITCHY SCALP-bergamot, tea tree, orange

DAMAGED, BLEACHED OR COLORED HAIR THAT NEEDS HEALING-sandalwood, ylang ylang, patchouli,

NORMAL HAIR THAT WANTS TO BE TREATED NATURALLY-geranium, lavender, ylang ylang

Additionaly we recommend you use herbal teas and supplements that contain aloe vera and clivers herb- these are excellent to prevent hair loss and stimulate hair growth.

Of course, it's not only about head and scalp massage. We suggest you use your massage time as time for reflection and meditation. Breathe in and out deeply. Massage your neck and your shoulders. Stretch intuitively and breathe in the wonderful and healing aromas.

You can also do it with your partner. It's really relaxing and therapeutic.

Below you will find a few recipes that we love using on a regular basis.

- **<u>Decongesting steam</u>**

While in the winter, some coughing and sniffles can be an irritant. Tea tree oil has powerful antiviral, combined with the potency of eucalyptus oil, which will help in decongesting the lungs and sinuses.

Ingredients
-4 cups boiling water
-5 drops eucalyptus essential oil (peppermint can also be used)
-5 drops tea tree essential oil

Process:

Boil the water in a teakettle. As soon as it comes to a boil, pour it into a large-enough container. Once this is done, mix the essential oils into it, and cover with a towel. Lift the towel and place your face so that your nose and mouth are only a few inches from the concoction. Take a couple of long and deep breaths, but make sure you spread a towel over your head.

Homemade Teething oil

Clove is a natural analgesic used in dentistry.

Ingredients

-2 tablespoons of olive oil, for a mild flavor 1 tablespoon of olive oil and 1 tablespoon of coconut oil.

-2-3 drops of clove bud essential oil

Process:

Combine the ingredients and taste it to make sure that it's not too strong. Then pour the mixture in a clean container. Since light oxidizes oil, use a dark amber container.

Use:

Make sure that the clove is absolutely diluted before application. Shake the mixture well and apply it on the gums with the fingertips. Reapply every 1-2 hours, as required.

Warming Chest Rub

Ingredients

-4 tsp Almond Oil

-4 tbsp Beeswax Pellets

-1 tbsp Coconut Butter

-30 drops Eucalyptus Oil

-10 drops Thyme Oil

-10 drops Tea Tree Oil

Process:

-In a glass bowl over boiling water, heat the almond oil, beeswax pellets, and coconut butter until melted. Remove the bowl from heat and let it sit for 60 seconds, keep stirring it to avoid solidification. Mix in essential oils, and pour them into a jar. Wait until the mixture has completely cooled before putting the cap on.

-When ready for use, rub a quarter sized portion between your fingers before placing on the child's (or your) chest or under the nose.

-Store this in a cool dark area for up to 1 month.

BONUS CHAPTER

DOSHA TEST

Hey, congratulations for going through his book to the very end.

Now, here comes the fan part- discovering yourself and learning more about your tendencies, strengths and weakness. This is really holistic stuff!

After doing this test you will know you prevalent dosha. Sometimes it might be even two doshas. Then, we suggest you start to observe your body, mind and emotions. If you want to take it to a new level, start your ayurvedic holistic diary.

Here's what you should include:

-How you feel today- your body, mind, feelings, emotions

-What body work have you done today

-What have you eaten

-Spices and herbs you have used

-Your spa treatments

This is how you will be able to notice certain patterns and emotions and how they influence your wellness. Once you discover that, you will be in the minority of Westerners who practice mindful and holistic self-care.

This process can also be abundant in errors. Don't worry about it. As long as you observe, learn and gradually eliminate negative habits from your lifestyle, you will be elbowing your way towards your health and wellbeing. Just like you have ever wanted!

For now just relax and do the test. Have a look which qualities prevail. This will be your prevalent dosha. Remember that no one is ever 100% vata, pitta or kapha. The tendencies and features mix and overlap. We also change and do our own holistic evolution.

Still, certain qualities are pre-born. For example some people are prone to colds, some people are prone to hair loss and some people are prone to weight gain. However, this does not mean that they should just sit with their arms crossed and not doing anything. Once should fight to at least try to improve their overall health. This is what oriental medicine is all about.

VATA

BODY TYPE- slim, light, fragile

HEIGHT-very tall or very short

WEIGHT-slim, light body weight. Veins and bones easily visible and marked.

SKIN-dry, sensitive, cold, sunburns easily

HAIR-dry, dandruff, very often brown or black

FACE-early wrinkles, small features,

EYES- small, dry, instable, dark

LIPS-slim, small, dry, can tremble easily

TEETH-small, there are spaces between them

CHEST-small, slim

HANDS- cold, dry, shaky. You can see veins and the bones mark easily.

NAILS-small, dry, cracked

FEET-large, dry, narrow

VOICE-speaks a lot, silent, soft, speaks fast

SLEEP-light, easily awaken, insomniac tendency

URINE-no color, does not urinate often

FECES- dry, easily constipated

PERSPIRATION-changeable, no strong odor, does not perspire a lot

APETITE-does not eat a lot, appetite changes depending on mood, when stressed does not eat

THIRST- changeable

CIRCULATION- poor, sluggish

ACTIVITY AND ENERGY-hyperactive, fast, likes to keep busy, very active

SENSITIVITY-hates cold, heat and wind

STAMINA AND STRENGTH-little stamina but can change, normally gets easily tired after excessive stamina workouts

DISEASES- TENDENCIES-arthritis, insomnia, nervousness, anxiety, mental imbalances

NEUROTIC TEMDEMCIES-anxiety, shakiness

POSITIVE MENTAL FEATURES-creative, active, enthusiastic, with imagination, motivating and motivated, encouraging, flexible

NEGATIVE MENTAL FEATURES-often in two minds, oversensitive, concerned about what other say.

SCORED....OUT OF 27

PITTA:

BODY TYPE- medium, quite strong

HEIGHT- medium

WEIGHT- medium, moderated, muscular

SKIN-red, humid, oily, beauty spots and freckles, can sun burn easily, can be prone to acne

HAIR-usually blonde or ginger, light colors. Quite thin and fragile. Prone to baldness and premature white hair.

FACE- reddish, tendency to get wrinkles on the forehead <but not always), very sharp features

EYES-light colors, sensitive, go read easily, penetrating, don't tolerate excess sun

LIPS-medium, red, soft

TEETH- medium, difficult to maintain them white (yellow tendencies), gums have tendency to bleed easily

CHEST-medium size

HANDS- warm, wet, medium, red

NAILS- have pinkish color, medium, soft

FEET-medium, soft, pinkish

VOICE-likes discussions and arguments, high-pitched, penetrating, strong

SLEEP- sleeps quite well but can wake up at night, usually able to get back to sleep again

URINE-abundant, yellow, red, warm

FECES- diarrhea tendency, goes to a bathroom a lot!

PERSPIRATION-abundant, strong odor, warm

APETITE- good digestion and excellent appetite, tends to overindulge in eating, drinking etc,

THIRST-strong, excessive, craves water all the time

CIRCULATION- strong, warm

ACTIVITY AND ENERGY- motivated, goal-orientated, with a plan to follow, well-organized, workaholic

SENSITIVITY-Fire, sun, heat- can't stand them, gets irritated

STAMINA AND STRENGTH-good stamina

DISEASES- TENDENCIES-fever, inflammation, infection

NEUROTIC TEMDEMCIES-anger, jealousy

POSITIVE MENTAL FEATURES-intelligent, competitive, very focused and centered

NEGATIVE MENTAL FEATURES- aggressive, irritable, easily frustrated

SCORED....OUT OF 27

KAPHA:

BODY TYPE- big, chubby, thick

HEIGHT-tall and husky or small and chubby

WEIGHT-excess weight

SKIN-arm, soft, oily, pale complexion

HAIR-wavy, curly, strong, fizzy, dark or light

FACE-big features, rounded

EYES-white, calm, attractive

LIPS-big, humid, firm

TEETH- white, big, strong

CHEST- big, strong

HANDS-big, oily, cold

NAILS-big, soft, white, strong

FEET-big, wide

VOICE-nice,- slow, does not talk a lot

SLEEP- hard to wake up!

URINE-white in color, moderate amounts

FECES-slow or moderate, solid

PERSPIRATION-moderate, cold

APETITE-uses food to escape from problems, if balanced, eats well, moderate amounts

THIRST does not drink too much

CIRCULATION- slow and steady

ACTIVITY AND ENERGY- slow, lazy, lethargic, can't motivate for action

SENSITIVITY-hates cold and humidity

STAMINA AND STRENGTH-good stamina, fit

DISEASES- TENDENCIES-water retention, overweight, respiratory system, runny nose

NEUROTIC TEMDEMCIES-does not feel like taking action, lethargic

POSITIVE MENTAL FEATURES-calm, steady, realistic

NEGATIVE MENTAL FEATURES- reluctant to change, stubborn, very sentimental

SCORED....OUT OF 27

Now do the math again...what's your prevalent dosha?

Conclusion

We have tried to provide you with the most pragmatic usage of Ayurvedic Aromatherapy so as to allow you to use their multiple combined benefits for a healthier and more energetic life. By using the methods described in this booklet, you can get started on aromatherapy in a holistic, Ayurvedic and personalized way.

Of course, this is only the beginning of your journey. We encourage you to study, explore and investigate and commit yourself to becoming a student of Ayurveda and gain a better and more balanced quality of life.

We hope that you are now on your way to discovering the multiple facets of Ayurvedic Aromatherapy and that you will be enjoying the immediate relief that it can provide you with!

You may also be interested in checking out our other book and learning more about Ayurveda and holistic healing:

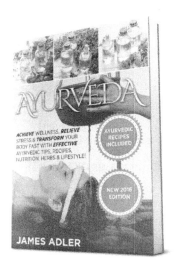

Available in your local Amazon Store

If you enjoyed our book and have a few seconds, please post your review. We would love to hear from you!

If you happen to have any questions or doubts or any kind of feedback for the next editions of this book, please send us an e-mail:

elenajamesbooks@gmail.com

Free Complimentary PDF eBook

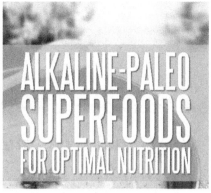

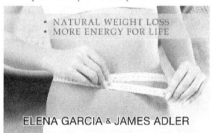

Download link:

www.bitly.com/alkapaleofree

Problems with your download?

Contact us: elenajamesbooks@gmail.com

Welcome to Holistic Wellness Books family!

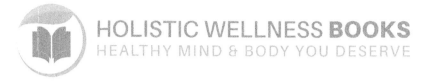

Follow us on Facebook & Twitter and be the first one to get free and bargain eBook and other holistic resources!

Click on the images below or visit:

www.twitter.com/Wellness_Books

www.facebook.com/HolisticWellnessBooks

Wishing you all the best on your Ayurvedic Aromatherapy journey!

Elena and James

www.amazon.com/author/elenagarcia

Made in the USA
Las Vegas, NV
27 November 2022

60444543R00066